Advances in Diagnostic Imaging
The Value of Contrast-Enhanced Ultrasound for Liver

Advances in Diagnostic Imaging

The Value of Contrast-Enhanced Ultrasound for Liver

Editor

Luigi Bolondi

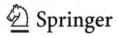 Springer

Editor
LUIGI BOLONDI
Division of Internal Medicine
Department of Internal Medicine
and Gastroenterology
University of Bologna, Italy

Authors
RICCARDO LENCIONI
CLOTILDE DELLA PINA
LAURA CROCETTI
DANIA CIONI
Division of Diagnostic
and Interventional Radiology
Department of Oncology,
Transplants, and Advanced
Technologies in Medicine
University of Pisa, Italy

HANS PETER WESKOTT
Department of Internal Medicine
Klinikum Hannover, Germany

JEAN-MICHEL CORREAS[1]
AHMED KHAIROUNE[1]
ANAIS VALLET-PICHARD[2]
STANISLAS POL[2]
OLIVIER HÉLÉNON[1]
Department of Adult Radiology[1]
and Department of Hepatology[2]
Necker University Hospital, Paris, France

ISBN-10   88-470-0457-8 Springer Milan Berlin Heidelberg New York

ISBN-13   978-88-470-0457-3 Springer Milan Berlin Heidelberg New York

Springer is a part of Springer Science+Business Media
springer.com
© Springer-Verlag Italia 2006

Cover design: Simona Colombo, Milan
Typesetting: Graficando, Milan

Introduction

It is well-known that, in the past few decades, imaging techniques, and in particular ultrasonography, have led to great advances in clinical hepatology. In fact, the widespread use of these techniques resulted in the clinical discovery of hepatocellular carcinoma and other liver tumours. Hepatocellular carcinoma was practically unknown to the clinician before the advent of diagnostic ultrasound. Real-time ultrasonography remains the most frequently used imaging procedure for the primary diagnosis of mass liver lesions and for the survey of patients affected by chronic liver diseases and tumours of the gastrointestinal tract.

In recent years, however, the imaging-based diagnosis of mass liver lesions has become increasingly complicated due to the number and morphological variability of lesions that modern imaging techniques are currently able to display. If the sensitivity in detection has greatly increased, characterization has remained difficult and represents a critical challenge for the clinician. In this perspective, the use of contrast agents with CT scan and MRI has represented a significant advance, allowing not only the depiction of different patterns of enhancement related to the different vascular supply of each lesion, but also to the detection of a higher number of lesions that become visible in different phases of vascular perfusion.

Hepatocellular carcinoma (HCC) most often displays a typical early arterial enhancement and a late washout of vascular contrast agents. This pattern, when confirmed by two different techniques, has been recognised by a panel of experts of the European Association for the Study of the Liver (EASL) as a valid criterion for the noninvasive diagnosis of HCC [1]. It is worth noting that duplex Doppler techniques are able to display some vascular abnormalities that characterise mass liver lesions; however, they are unable to display different phases of perfusion and have a overall sensitivity far less than that of contrast-enhanced CT and MRI.

The availability of blood-pool contrast agents for ultrasound (US) together with the development of US harmonic imaging has opened up new perspectives both for the immediate characterization of any mass lesion detected in the liver and for increasing the sensitivity of ultrasonography in the detection of liver metastases. The technique was initially based on digital processing of nonlinear backscattered signals produced by the breaking of first-generation microbubble contrast agents when insonated by high acoustic pressure [mechanical index (MI) = 0.8–1.2] US waves. Nevertheless, since these microbubbles are destroyed by the high pressure, a certain amount of time (depending on the blood perfusion velocity in the explored tissue) must elapse to allow refilling of the microvessels by the contrast agent. As a result, signals originating from microbubble destruction must be explored by an intermittent imaging modality. This method is technically complicated, affected by artefacts, and does not allow continuous dynamic evaluation of vascular perfusion. In addition, at high acoustic pressure, harmonic signals may be also produced by the surrounding tissue, thus limiting the contrast resolution of the image.

More recently, contrast-specific software and technologies have been developed that facilitate the analysis of harmonic signals originating from the insonation of second-generation US contrast agents by using extremely low acoustic pressure (MI = 0.04–0.1) US waves. These second-generation contrast agents are based on the more stable perfluorocarbon-filled or sulfur-hexafluoride-filled microbubbles and have a strong nonlinear harmonic response when insonated with low acoustic pressure. A second-generation blood pool agent, BR1 (SonoVue; Bracco, Milan, Italy), consisting of phospholipid-stabilised shell microbubbles filled with sulfur hexafluoride gas, is licensed for use in abdominal and vascular imaging in most European countries. The safety and effectiveness of this agent have been proved in preliminary experimental and clinical investigations. New US technologies avoid microbubble destruction and allow continuous real-time imaging of the liver parenchyma and of liver tumours during vascular perfusion. For this reason, the technique is also referred to as "perfusional angiosonography", in order to distinguish it from techniques using first-generation contrast agents and intermittent imaging. Several contrast-specific US modes operating at low acoustic pressure have been introduced in clinical practice.

Taking into account the great impact of this new technology on clinical practice, the European Federation of Societies for Ultrasound in Medicine and Biology (EFSUMB) organised, in January 2004, in Rotterdam, a consensus meeting of experts in order to develop guidelines for the use of US contrast agents in the diagnosis of liver diseases [2]. The resulting document represents an important starting point for clinical implementation of this new diagnostic procedure. The guidelines as well as further advances in the clinical application of contrast-enhanced harmonic US were presented by a group of the experts (JM Correas, R Lencioni and HP Weskott) from the Rotterdam meeting at the Bracco satellite symposium, held in Paris in April 2005 during the annual EASL congress, and are reported in this booklet. Finally, in June 2005 a panel of experts from EASL, the American Association for the Study of the Liver (AASLD), and the Japanese Society of Hepatology (JSH) met at the EASL monothematic conference in Barcelona. This group reviewed both the data available in the literature and the body of clinical experience that has resulted from different eastern and western countries. The panel introduced contrast-enhanced harmonic US among the techniques able to provide specific findings for the diagnosis of HCC.

The implementation of these guidelines will result in a considerable increase in the request for contrast-enhanced US procedures. Consequently, US services will have to update their equipment, provide proper training to physicians performing US examinations, and take into account the cost of introduction of these procedures into daily practice. Whether the eventual cost saving associated with reduced demand for CT or MR imaging of the liver after contrast-enhanced US largely counterbalances the cost of the examination should be investigated by a pharmaco-economical analysis.

Luigi Bolondi
Division of Internal Medicine
Department of Internal Medicine
and Gastroenterology
University of Bologna, Italy

▉ References

1. Bruix J, Sherman M, Llovet JM et al (2001) EASL Panel of Experts on HCC. Clinical management of hepatocellular carcinoma. Conclusions of the Barcelona-2000 EASL conference. European Association for the Study of the Liver. J Hepatol 35: 421-430
2. Albrecht T, Blomley M, Bolondi L et al; EFSUMB Study Group (2004) Guidelines for the use of contrast agents in ultrasound. Ultraschall Med 25:249-256

Contents

RICCARDO LENCIONI, CLOTILDE DELLA PINA,
LAURA CROCETTI, DANIA CIONI

Chapter 1

Impact of European Federation of Societies for Ultrasound in Medicine and Biology (EFSUMB) Guidelines on the Use of Contrast Agents in Liver Ultrasound

Riccardo Lencioni, Clotilde Della Pina,
Laura Crocetti, Dania Cioni
Division of Diagnostic and Interventional Radiology
Department of Oncology, Transplants,
and Advanced Technologies in Medicine
University of Pisa, Italy

Introduction

The detection and characterization of focal liver lesions is an important and challenging issue. Hepatocellular carcinoma (HCC) is the fifth most common cancer [1]. The liver is the organ most frequently involved by metastases from other tumors. In addition, benign liver lesions, such as hemangioma and focal nodular hyperplasia (FNH), have a high prevalence in the general population. Several imaging modalities and diagnostic protocols have been used in attempts to optimize detection and characterization of focal liver lesions.

Ultrasound (US) is the most commonly used liver imaging modality worldwide. Unfortunately, it has limited sensitivity in the detection of small tumor nodules. Moreover, US findings are often nonspecific, as there are enough variability and overlap in the appearances of benign and malignant liver lesions to make a definite distinction problematic. Computed tomography (CT) and magnetic resonance (MR) imaging are commonly used to clarify questionable US findings and to provide a more comprehensive assessment of the liver parenchyma.

Recently, the introduction of microbubble contrast agents and the development of contrast-specific techniques have opened new prospects in liver US [2]. Contrast-specific techniques produce images based on nonlinear acoustic effects of microbubbles and display enhancement in gray-scale, maximizing contrast, and spatial resolution. The goal of improving the US assessment of focal lesions was initially pursued by scanning the liver with high mechanical index (MI) techniques, in which the signal is produced by the collapse of the microbubbles. The main limitations of this destructive method is that it produces a transient display of the contrast agent. Thus, it requires intermittent scanning, and a series of sweeps are needed to cover the whole liver parenchyma. The advent of second-generation agents – which have higher harmonic emission capabilities – has been instrumental in improving the ease and reproducibility of the examination [3]. In fact, a lower, nondestructive MI can be used, thus enabling continuous real-time imaging. Over the past few years, several reports have shown that real-time contrast-enhanced US can substantially improve detection and characterization of focal liver lesions with respect to baseline studies [4].

With the publication of guidelines for the use of contrast agents in liver US by the European Federation of Societies for Ultrasound in Medicine and Biology (EFSUMB), contrast-enhanced US has entered into clinical practice [4]. The guidelines define the indications and recommendations for the use of contrast agents in focal liver lesion detection, characterization, and post-treatment follow-up. In this chapter, the impact of EFSUMB guidelines on the diagnostic protocols currently adopted in liver imaging is discussed with regard to four clinical scenarios: (1) characterization of focal liver lesions of incidental detection; (2) diagnosis of HCC in patients with cirrhosis; (3) detection of hepatic metastases in oncology patients; and (4) guidance and assessment of the outcome of percutaneous tumor ablation procedures.

Characterization of Incidental Focal Liver Lesions

Characterization of focal lesions of incidental detection is one of the most common and sometimes troublesome issues in liver imaging. Unsuspected lesions, in fact, are frequently detected in patients who have neither chronic liver disease nor a history of malignancy during an US examination of the abdomen. While a confident diagnosis is usually made on the basis of US findings in cases of simple cysts and hemangiomas with typical hyperechoic appearance, lesions with nonspecific US features require further investigation [5]. The patient is typically referred for contrast-enhanced CT or contrast-enhanced MR imaging of the liver.

EFSUMB guidelines recommend the use of contrast agents to diagnose benign focal lesions not characterized at baseline study. This statement is based on the ability of contrast US to carefully analyze lesion vascularity. In fact, lesions that most frequently cause incidental findings, i.e., hemangioma and FNH, typically show contrast-enhanced US patterns that closely resemble those at contrast-enhanced CT or contrast-enhanced MR imaging. Most liver hemangiomas show peripheral nodular enhancement during the early phase, with progressive centripetal fill-in leading to lesion hyperchogenicity in the late phase (Fig. 1). In two recent series, this characteristic features was shown in 78-93% of hemangiomas [6, 7]. FNH presents as a central vascular supply with centrifugal filling in the early arterial phase, followed by homogeneous enhancement in the late arterial phase. In the portal phase, the lesion remains hyperechoic relative to normal liver tissue and becomes isoechoic in the late phase (Fig. 2). This pattern has been observed in 85-100% of FNHs [6, 8]. Therefore, it appears that in most liver lesions incidentally discovered at the baseline US study, detection of typical enhancement patterns after contrast injection may enable a quick and confident diagnosis, possibly avoiding the need for more complex and expensive investigations.

Fig. 1a-h. Hemangioma. At baseline ultrasound (US), the lesion has atypical features and appears as an iso/hypoechoic nodule (**a**). At contrast-enhanced US, the lesion shows peripheral nodular enhancement in the arterial phase (**b**) with centripetal filling in the portal-venous and delayed phases (**c, d**). The enhancement pattern resembles that observed at multidetector computed tomography CT. **e** Baseline, **f** Arterial phase, **g** Portal-venous phase, **h** Delayed phase

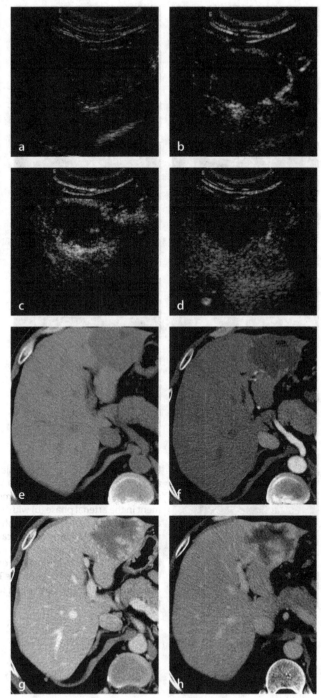

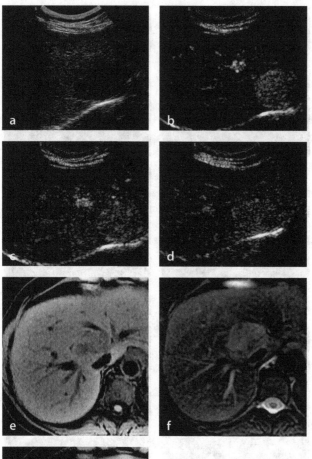

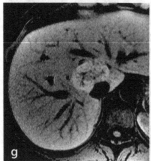

Fig. 2a-g. Focal nodular hyperplasia. Baseline US shows a hypoechoic lesion on segment VIII (**a**). At contrast-enhanced US, the lesion shows homogeneous enhancement in the arterial phase (**b**) with an isoechoic appearance in the portal and delayed phases (**c, d**). At magnetic resonance (MR) imaging, focal nodular hyperplasia appears slightly hypointense on the T1-weighted image (**e**), slightly hyperintense on the T2-weighted image (**f**), and hyperintense on the T1-weighted image acquired 1 h after injection of an hepatospecific contrast agent (**g**)

Diagnosis of Hepatocellular Carcinoma in Cirrhosis

The second clinical scenario is that of patients with hepatic cirrhosis. In view of the high risk to develop HCC, these patients are carefully followed with US examinations repeated at 6-month intervals [9]. While the detection of a focal lesion in cirrhosis should always raise the suspicion of HCC, it is well-established that the pathologic changes inherent in cirrhosis may simulate HCC in a variety of ways, especially because nonmalignant hepatocellular lesions, such as regenerative and dysplastic nodules, may be indistinguishable from a small tumor. One of the key pathologic factors for differential diagnosis that is reflected in imaging appearances is the vascular supply to the nodule. Through the progression from regenerative nodule to dysplastic nodule to frank HCC, there is loss of visualization of portal tracts and development of new arterial vessels, termed nontriadal arteries, which become the dominant blood supply in overt HCC. It is this neovascularity that allows HCC to be diagnosed with contrast-enhanced CT or dynamic MR imaging [10].

According to EFSUMB guidelines, carrying out a contrast-enhanced US study is recommended to characterize any lesion or suspect lesion detected at baseline US in the setting of liver cirrhosis [4]. Owing to the ability to display contrast enhancement in real-time, contrast US provides a tool to show arterial neoangiogenesis associated with malignant change, and therefore to help establish the diagnosis of HCC [11, 12]. HCC typically shows strong intratumoral enhancement in the arterial phase (i.e., within 25-35 s after the start of contrast injection) followed by rapid wash-out with an isoechoic or hypoechoic appearance in the portal-venous and delayed phases (Fig. 3). In contrast, neither a large regenerative nodule nor dysplastic nodules usually show any early contrast uptake, but instead resemble the enhancement pattern of liver parenchyma. Selective arterial enhancement at contrast US has been observed in 91-96% of HCC lesions, confirming that contrast US may be a tool to show arterial neoangiogenesis of HCC [11, 12]. In a recent study, in which findings at spiral CT were assumed as the gold standard, the sensitivity of

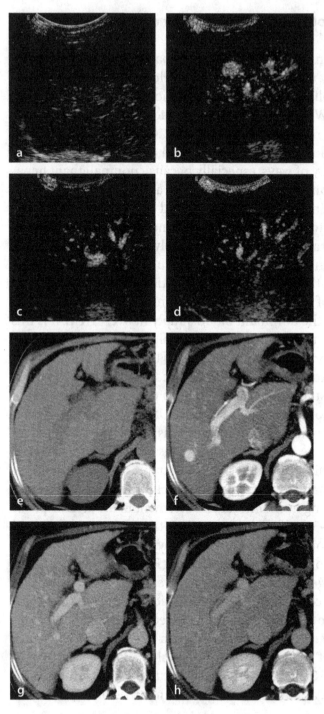

Fig. 3a-h. Hepatocellular carcinoma. At baseline US examination, the lesion appears as an iso/hypoechoic nodule (**a**). At contrast-enhanced US, the lesion shows early enhancement in the arterial phase (**b**) with rapid wash-out in the portal-venous and delayed phases (**c, d**). By multidetector CT the same enhancement pattern is observed. **e** Baseline, **f** Arterial phase, **g** Portal-venous phase, **h** Delayed phase contrast US in the detection of arterial hypervascularity was 97% in lesions > 3 cm, 92% in lesions ranging 2-3 cm, 87% in lesions ranging 1-2 cm, and 67% in lesions < 1 cm [12]. Hence, a contrast-enhanced study is recommended in all lesions or suspected lesions ≥ 1 cm in diameter that are detected at baseline US in cirrhosis or chronic hepatitis patients participating in surveillance programs.

Detection of Hepatic Metastases in Oncology Patients

Metastatic disease involving the liver is one of the most common issues in oncology. CT and positron emission tomography (PET) are used in oncology protocols to provide objective documentation of the extent of the liver tumor burden and to effectively assess extrahepatic disease. Nevertheless, US is widely used in post-treatment follow-up to monitor tumor response and to detect the emergence of new hepatic metastatic lesions. One of the major points addressed by the EFSUMB document is the use of contrast agents in this patient population. In fact, the use of contrast agents is recommended not only to clarify a questionable lesion detected at baseline examination; rather, a contrast-enhanced ultrasound study is recommended in every oncology patients referred for liver US, unless clear-cut disseminated disease is detected at the baseline study. This means that all liver US examinations conducted to rule out liver metastases should include a contrast-enhanced study, even if the baseline scans do not show any abnormality. This strong statement is based on the substantial increase in the ability to detect liver metastases in contrast-enhanced studies compared to baseline [13]. Even small metastases stand out as markedly hypoechoic lesions against the enhanced liver parenchyma throughout the portal-venous and delayed phases (Fig. 4). The earlier the detection of liver metastatic disease, the earlier the therapeutic intervention.

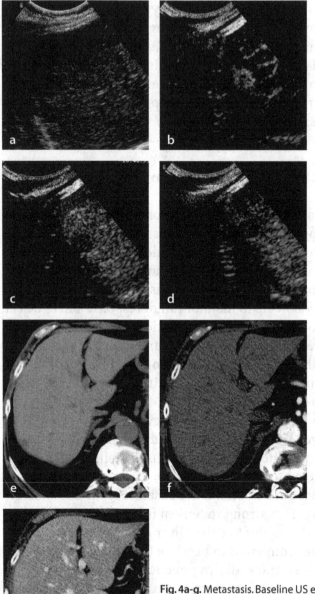

Fig. 4a-g. Metastasis. Baseline US examination shows a subcapsular hypoechoic nodule (**a**). At contrast-enhanced US, the lesion shows rim enhancement during the arterial phase (**b**), with a hypoechoic appearance in the portal-venous and delayed phases (**c, d**). By multidetector CT, the metastatic nodule appears hypodense in the baseline scan (**e**) as well as in the arterial (**f**) and delayed (**g**) phases

Guidance and Monitoring of Tumor Ablation Procedures

Several percutaneous techniques have been developed to treat nonsurgical patients with liver malignancies. These minimally invasive procedures can achieve effective and reproducible tumor destruction with acceptable morbidity. Radiofrequency ablation is increasingly accepted as the best therapeutic choice for patients with early-stage HCC when resection or transplantation are precluded, and it has also become a viable treatment approach for patients with limited hepatic metastatic disease from colorectal cancer who are not eligible for surgical resection [14, 15].

When US is used as the imaging modality for guiding ablations, the addition of contrast agent can provide additional important information throughout all procedural steps: (a) it improves delineation and conspicuity of lesions poorly visualized on baseline scans, facilitating targeting; (b) it allows immediate assessment of treatment outcome by showing the disappearance of any previously visualized intralesional enhancement; (c) it may be useful in follow-up protocols for early detection of tumor recurrence [16].

Conclusions

Despite the improvement in detection and characterization of focal liver lesions that can be achieved by using contrast-enhanced US, several issues remain to be resolved. First, contrast US will hardly replace CT or MR imaging for preoperative assessment of patients with liver tumors, as these techniques still offer a more comprehensive assessment of the liver parenchyma, which is mandatory to properly plan any kind of surgical or interventional procedure. Second, the daily schedule of each US laboratory doing liver examinations will have to be reformulated, and many such laboratories will have to update their equipment and provide proper training for their doctors. Last but not least, the cost of the introduction of contrast-enhanced US into daily practice will have to be taken into account. It can be argued that cost savings associated with patients who will no longer need CT or MR imaging of the liver after contrast-enhanced US could largely counterbalance the cost of the examination. However, an optimal use of contrast-enhanced US will require precise diagnostic flow charts for each clinical situation. Nevertheless, contrast-enhanced US has the potential to become the primary liver-imaging modality for early detection and characterization of focal lesions. Early diagnosis of primary and secondary liver malignancies greatly enhances the possibility of curative surgical resection or successful percutaneous ablation, resulting in better patient care and eventually in improved patient survival.

References

1. Llovet JM, Burroughs A, Bruix J (2003) Hepatocellular carcinoma. Lancet 362:1907-1917
2. Lencioni R, Cioni D, Bartolozzi C (2002) Tissue harmonic and contrast-specific imaging: back to gray scale in ultrasound. Eur Radiol 12:151-165
3. Lencioni R, Cioni D, Crocetti L et al (2002) Ultrasound imaging of focal liver lesions with a second-generation contrast agent. Acad Radiol 9(Suppl 2):371-374
4. Albrecht T, Blomley M, Bolondi L et al; EFSUMB Study Group (2004) Guidelines for the use of contrast agents in ultrasound. January 2004. Ultraschall Med 25:249-256
5. Lencioni R, Cioni D, Crocetti L et al (2004) Magnetic resonance imaging of liver tumors. J Hepatol 40:162-171
6. Wen YL, Kudo M, Zheng RQ et al (2004) Characterization of hepatic tumors: value of contrast-enhanced coded phase-inversion harmonic angio. AJR Am J Roentgenol 182:1019-1026
7. Quaia E, Calliada F, Bertolotto M et al (2004) Characterization of focal liver lesions with contrast-specific US modes and a sulfur hexafluoride-filled microbubble contrast agent: diagnostic performance and confidence. Radiology 232:420-430
8. Kim MJ, Lim HK, Kim SH et al (2004) Evaluation of hepatic focal nodular hyperplasia with contrast-enhanced gray scale harmonic sonography: initial experience. J Ultrasound Med 23:297-305

9. Bruix J, Sherman M, Llovet JM et al; EASL Panel of Experts on HCC (2001) Clinical management of hepatocellular carcinoma. Conclusions of the Barcelona-2000 EASL conference. European Association for the Study of the Liver. J Hepatol 35:421-430

10. Lencioni R, Cioni D, Della Pina C et al (2005) Imaging diagnosis. Semin Liver Dis 25:162-170

11. Nicolau C, Catala V, Vilana R et al (2004) Evaluation of hepatocellular carcinoma using SonoVue, a second generation ultrasound contrast agent: correlation with cellular differentiation. Eur Radiol 14:1092-1099

12. Gaiani S, Celli N, Piscaglia F et al (2004) Usefulness of contrast-enhanced perfusional sonography in the assessment of hepatocellular carcinoma hypervascular at spiral computed tomography. J Hepatol 41:421-426

13. Oldenburg A, Hohmann J, Foert E et al (2005) Detection of hepatic metastases with low MI real time contrast enhanced sonography and SonoVue. Ultraschall Med 26:277-284

14. Lencioni R, Crocetti L, Cioni D et al (2004) Percutaneous radiofrequency ablation of hepatic colorectal metastases. Technique, indications, results, and new promises. Invest Radiol 39:689-697

15. Lencioni R, Cioni D, Crocetti L et al (2005) Early-stage hepatocellular carcinoma in patients with cirrhosis: long-term results of percutaneous image-guided radiofrequency ablation. Radiology 234:961-967

16. Solbiati L, Ierace T, Tonolini M, Cova L (2004) Guidance and monitoring of radiofrequency liver tumor ablation with contrast-enhanced ultrasound. Eur J Radiol 51(Suppl):19-23

Hans Peter Weskott

Chapter 2

The Role of Contrast-Enhanced Ultrasound (CEUS) in Identifying and Characterizing Focal Liver Lesions

Hans Peter Weskott
Department of Internal Medicine
Klinikum Hannover, Germany

Introduction

Differences in the acoustic properties of tumor and liver tissue are the basis for B-mode ultrasound (US), which is used for the detection and characterization of focal liver lesions (FLL). The ability of US to discriminate between normal and abnormal liver tissue is limited: Compared to contrast-enhanced computed tomography (CT), magnetic resonance imaging (MRI), or positron emission tomography (PET), unenhanced gray scale US has the lowest detection rate for FLLs.

Contrast agents have been commercially available in most European countries since 1996. The second-generation contrast agent SonoVue (Bracco, Italy), available since 2001, consists of bubbles that have a flexible shell, allowing them to oscillate when insonated at low acoustic power [so-called low mechanical index (MI) imaging mode]. These resonating bubbles generate harmonic echo frequencies that can constantly be imaged in a real-time fashion. Low MI imaging technique using a second-generation contrast agent (SonoVue) has become the method of choice for detection and characterization of FLL.

Although contrast agents can be used in the diagnostic work-up of many organs, the greatest progress has been made in diagnosing liver diseases. The main diagnostic goals are tumor detection and characterization. Both can excellently be achieved by visual interpretation of the contrast study. Long digitally stored loops can either be reviewed online at the time of the examination or later, either from the US machine's memory or offline at the workstation.

Examination Technique

Prior to contrast-enhanced ultrasound (CEUS), a conventional unenhanced US baseline examination is performed, including tissue harmonic and color flow imaging techniques. The latter may already show a tumor-supplying vessel or intra-tumoral vessels, which helps to optimize the scanning position for the following CEUS. A sweep done in gray-scale technique aims at the detection of FLL and at finding the best examination position.

The optimal MI number depends on the scanning conditions and US device used. For most US devices, it ranges between 0.08 and 0.20. With increasing MI numbers, the percentage of destroyed bubbles will increase. A Sonovue bolus of 1.0-4.8 ml – in most cases 2.4 ml – is injected intravenously, followed by a 10-ml saline flush.

The dual blood supply of the liver makes this organ unique and hemodynamic studies challenging. About 70% of the total volume blood supply (about 1500 ml/min = 20% of the cardiac output) comes from the portal vein, the remainder from the hepatic artery. Microbubbles can trespass the capillary beds without being destroyed and can thus enhance vessels and organs like the abdominal organs or the brain. The microbubbles (air or gas) are eliminated in the lungs, the shell and stabilizing agents in the liver. US contrast agents are strictly intravascular and do not enhance the interstitium, unlike CT and MR contrast media. US contrast agent does not appear in the biliary system or the urinary tract. The dynamic changes in contrast enhancement of the liver over time are characterized by different phases (Table 1).

Table 1. Characterization of contrast phases of the liver

Phase	Visualization post-injection time	
	Start (s)	End (s)
Arterial phase	10-20	25-35
Portal-venous phase	30-45	120
Late phase	>120	Bubble disappearance

Contrast kinetics, that is, the arrival times of bubbles in the hepatic artery, portal vein, and liver veins, and the duration of contrast phases depend on global hemodynamic changes and can therefore be modulated in patients with heart failure.

The blood supply of malignant liver lesions is nearly completely provided by arteries, and arteriovenous shunts are frequently present, the wash-out in most liver metastases being much quicker than in normal liver parenchyma. Benign solid lesions often can be best detected and characterized during the wash-in phase of the contrast agent and vanish in later phases.

In order to detect as many benign and malignant lesions as possible, a sweep during the arterial phase is recommended, as the tumor vasculature can be best studied during the wash-in phase of the contrast agent, since the enhancement level between normal liver tissue and solid benign lesions after the wash-in phase will not differ in most cases. The sweep should start with the advent of the bubbles into the major arterial branches. As in the baseline study, during CEUS it is mandatory to perform a sweep of the liver tissue that covers both liver lobes completely, while during the portal-venous (PV) and late phases liver tissue should be imaged in a longitudinal and cross-sectional scan plane. As the arterial phase lasts for only 10 to maximum 20 s, a second bolus might be necessary for the examination of both liver lobes.

For tumor characterization, a continuous scanning of at least one reference lesion in a scan plane allows the arrival, filling up, and wash-out of contrast material to be monitored in a real-time fashion. In hypervascular lesions, a high MI burst performed between the mid- and late arterial phases may again demonstrate arterial refilling of the lesion. All cine loops should be digitally recorded and reviewed stepwise at the end of the examination. Prior to a follow-up study, the latest contrast examinations have to be reviewed in order to make the scanning conditions and the settings of the US device comparable.

The change of signal intensity in a region of interest can be analyzed from video or, better, from the raw data (TIC, time intensity curve) (Fig. 6, and see Fig. 15). Three-dimensional rendering often gives a better idea of the number and location of the tumor-supplying vessels.

Indications

Indications for the examination of the liver range from a general check-up to clinical signs of liver disease or the risk of developing liver metastasis or hepatocellular carcinoma (HCC). In the follow-up of tumor patients, the biggest challenge is monitoring malignant lesions, especially in patients receiving chemotherapy (Fig. 1). It is well-known that chemotherapy changes the echogenicity of both liver tissue and the targeted lesions; as a result, US studies may be misleading [1].

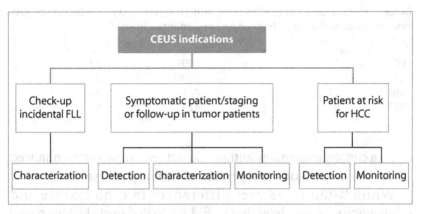

Fig. 1. Indications for the use of second-generation contrast agent in suspected focal liver lesions and diagnostic work-up. *FLL* = focal liver lesions, *HCC* = hepatocellular carcinoma

CEUS in the Detection of FLL

In pathological-anatomic studies, incidentally found FLLs exceed 50% [2]. Among these, hemangiomas represent the largest group (up to 20%), while focal nodular hyperplasia account for 3%. Due to the widespread use of US, hemangiomas are incidentally found in about 7-8% of patients. Small liver tumors detected in asymptomatic patients are most likely benign, especially lesions < 15 mm [3], even in patients with known malignancies.

Beside differences in the acoustic appearance of benign vs. malignant lesions, a lesion has to reach a certain size to make it detectable. Some 30% of all liver metastases are < 10 mm, as determined in patients receiving the best-available reference imaging technique (intra-operative US). For every metastasis in colorectal cancer exceeding 10 mm, 1.6 metastases were found to be smaller than 10 mm, and up to a 4 fold number of other primary tumors, such as breast cancer. By contrast, only 20% of FLL < 15 mm are malignant in patients with known cancers [4]. Therefore, after detection of FLLs, their characterization is most important, with small lesions being the most challenging.

Before the era of US contrast media, the sensitivity of gray-scale US in detecting FLL was poor compared to other imaging modalities [5] (Table 2).

Table 2. Meta-analysis of studies comparing the sensitivity in detection of liver metastases of malignant intestinal tumors (adapted from [4])

	Number of data sets	Patients	Sensitivity (%)
US	11	509	55
CT	25	1,747	72
MR	11	401	76
PET	9	423	90

As a consequence many authors do not recommend un-enhanced US for the diagnostic management of tumor patients [1, 6].

While B-mode US uses differences in echo texture and echogenicity for the detection of FLLs, CEUS detects lesions based on their different enhancement levels or patterns during the different phases. The detection rate for FLL depends on the imaging technique and individual scanning conditions and on the size and degree of vascularization as well.

Depending on differences in vascularity, the detection rate of the various tumor entities may differ. The highest sensitivity in detecting both benign and malignant lesions is obtained by continuous observation of the contrast kinetics over all phases. Both B-mode US and CEUS have biological and technical limitations, such as inadequate access to the liver, high tissue attenuation, and a limited spatial resolution. Detection of the smallest lesions by CEUS depends on the spatial resolution of the US system, attenuation, and depth of the lesion. It usually ranges between 3 and 4 mm.

Additionally, it is mandatory to detect as many lesions as possible. Many CEUS studies found an increase in the number of detected liver metastases compared to unenhanced examinations and a comparable number compared to spiral CT. In patients with resectable colorectal liver metastases found by spiral CT scans, additional liver metastases were found intra-operatively by US in 30% of patients [7]. Recently, Konopke reported an increase in the number of detected lesions from 53% (B-mode) to 86% (CEUS) prior to laparoscopic examination [8].

While a combination of B-mode US and the arterial phase seem to detect most benign FLL, the PV and late phases are the most important for the detection of malignant lesions. In a minority of patients, and in some cases of highly differentiated hypervascular metastases, the arterial phase may be more sensitive. In a CT study, Paulson [9] found that one sixth of carcinoid metastases are only detectable during the arterial phase.

Characterization of FLL

It is well-known that B-mode US, including the use of color flow imaging techniques, is deficient with respect to tumor characterization. The assessment of tumor vascularity is believed to add important information. The basis for characterization a lesion by means of CEUS is comparison between the enhancement level of a focal lesion and the normal liver parenchyma during all three contrast phases. As tumor and liver tissue differ in contrast uptake, distribution, and wash-out, all three phases are needed to classify a tumor. During the arterial phase, the size, number, and architecture of tumor vascularity can be studied. Arterial enhancement in malignant lesions may last only briefly, and since the following PV and late phases may already demonstrate a wash-out, the arterial phase often provides the most useful information for characterizing a lesion – especially benign ones. During PV phase and in some cases lasting into the late phase, the intralesional distribution of enhanced tumor tissue may differ in terms of homogeneity. Another criterion for characterization is the direction of intralesional enhancement over time (Fig. 2).

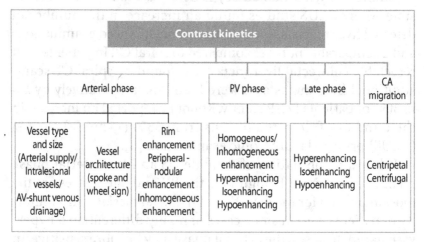

Fig. 2. Diagnostic criteria during all three phased of contrast enhancement. *PV* = portalvenous, *CA* = contrast agent

Differentiation of Benign and Malignant Liver Lesions

After detection of a lesion, criteria have to be established to differentiate benign from malignant lesions. B-mode US lacks specificity in characterizing FLLs; its specificity in differentiating between benign and malignant ranges between 23 and 68% on baseline study. Color and spectral Doppler are limited in the detection of tiny vessels and/or low-flow states in all FLL [10].

Preoperative MR and intra-operative US are much more reliable, but may also fail: Sahani reported that in 250 consecutive patients undergoing hepatic resection for presumed malignancy, 18 (7.2%) were shown to have lesions with benign pathology. Compared to intra-operative US, pre-operative MR failed to identify 7.5% lesions and 5.6% were not detected by either method [11].

The gold standard for tissue characterization is histology. The role of fine-needle biopsies has to be questioned, as the sensitivity of fine-needle aspiration cytology (FNAC) for detecting hepatic malignancy has been reported to be 90-93% [12, 13], thus being similar to the diagnostic accuracy obtainable with radiological investigations, including CEUS, which have up to > 90% sensitivity [14, 15]. Furthermore, biopsy of hepatic adenomas, focal nodular hyperplasia, and hemangiomas also carries an increased bleeding risk.

The persistent enhancement of FLL compared to normal liver parenchyma in the late phase is the most important criterion to differentiate between benign and malignant lesions: With the exception of cysts and completely thrombosed hemangiomas (Fig. 3), all benign lesions can be characterized during the late phase as isoenhancing or slightly hyperenhancing when com-

Fig. 3. Completely thrombosed hemangioma (confirmed by MRI). No enhancement could be detected at any of the three phases. **a** Baseline, **b** Arterial phase, **c** PV phase, **d** Late phase

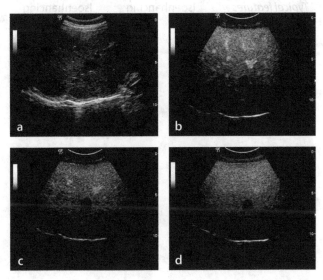

pared to surrounding normal liver tissue. When applying this criterion to FLLs, the specificity of this sign ranges between 95 and 100% [14, 16-18].

Benign Lesions

The most common benign FLL are hepatic cysts, hemangiomas, focal nodular hyperplasia (FNH), focal fatty sparing, focal hepatic steatosis, and regenerative nodules. Even the majority of lesions < 15 mm found in patients with a history of extrahepatic malignancy are benign in 89% of cases [4]. All focal areas containing normal liver tissue enhance like the surrounding liver tissue. Regenerative nodules may slightly differ in their vascular supply and may thus hyper- or hypoenhance during the arterial phase (Fig. 2).

Focal Fatty Changes

As an area of focal fatty infiltration or fatty sparing does not differ in its vasculature from surrounding liver tissue, contrast enhancement does not differ as well from surrounding tissue (Table 3).

Table 3. Characteristic features in circumscriptive fatty sparing and focal steatosis (from [19])

Tumor entity	Arterial phase	PV phase	Delayed (late) phase
Typical features	Isoenhancing	Isoenhancing	Isoenhancing

Liver Cysts

The diagnosis of liver cysts in B-mode US can be confirmed by CEUS. Hepatic cysts do not enhance at any time after contrast injection. As in B-mode, US an enhancement of liver tissue distal from the cyst may occur (Fig. 4).

In case a suspected cyst is first detected during late phase, switching to a high MI imaging mode will demonstrate again the typical gray-scale signs of a cyst.

A rim enhancement around a cyst may be a sign of inflammation or of a malignant lesion (Fig. 5).

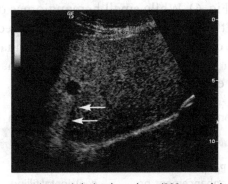

Fig. 4. Cystic enhancement (*arrows*) during late phase (283s post-injection)

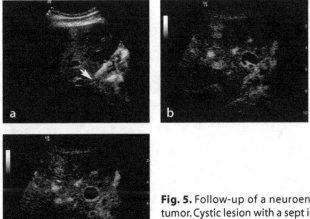

Fig. 5. Follow-up of a neuroendrocrine pancreatic tumor. Cystic lesion with a sept in segment VI (*arrow*), enhancement of the wall and sept. Metastasis was confirmed by biopsy. **a** Baseline, **b** Arterial phase, **c** Arterial phase

Hemangioma

Incidentally detected FLL in asymptomatic patients are by far most likely benign. It is therefore not surprising that, even in nonenhanced US studies, lesions can be characterized with a high reliability: Hemangiomas with typical B-mode appearance [20] in asymptomatic patients can be correctly diagnosed in nearly all cases [21]. However, in patients at risk for HCC, the same B-mode criteria may fail to characterize hemangiomas in half of the cases [22]. Hemangiomas are uncommon in cirrhotic livers [23].

The most typical feature in hemangioma is an early peripheral nodular enhancement with a progressive centripetal filling [24] (Table 4, Fig. 6). While small hemangiomas often fill completely during the arterial or early PV phase, especially in larger hemangiomas central areas often remain unenhanced (thrombosed vascular channels) (Figs. 7, 8). Some hemangiomas may hyperenhance even until late phase (Figs. 9, 10).

Table 4. CEUS characteristics of hepatic hemangiomas (from [19])

Tumor entity	Arterial phase	PV phase	Delayed (late) phase
Typical features	Peripheral-nodular enhancement, no central enhancement	Partial/complete centripetal filling	Complete enhancement
Additional features	Small lesions: complete, rapid centripetal enhancement		Nonenhancing central areas

Fig. 6. Typical contrast kinetics of a hemangioma. Peripheral nodular enhancement in the arterial phase, followed by a centripetal filling. The quick rise in signal intensity on the time-intensity curve (*TIC*) demonstrates the arterial character of the supplying peripheral vessels. **a** Arterial phase (12s), **b** PV phase (65s), **c** Late phase (144s), **d** TIC

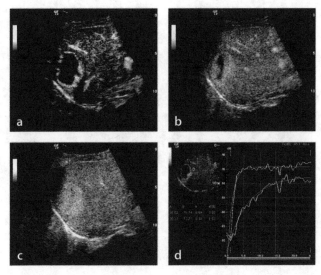

Fig. 7. Typical contrast kinetics of a 6-cm hemangioma. Even during late phase, the center is not completely enhanced. **a** Baseline, **b** Arterial phase (15s), **c** PV phase (62s), **d** Late phase (121s)

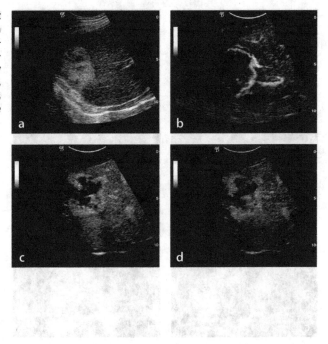

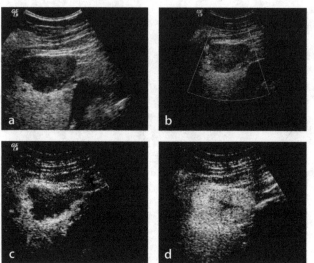

Fig. 8. Atypical echo-poor B-mode appearance of a hemangioma in a patient with prostate cancer. Typical contrast kinetics. Note the central scar-like contrast defect, which might be misleading for focal nodular hyperplasia. **a** Baseline, **b** CDI image, **c** Arterial phase (16s), **d** PV phase (61s)

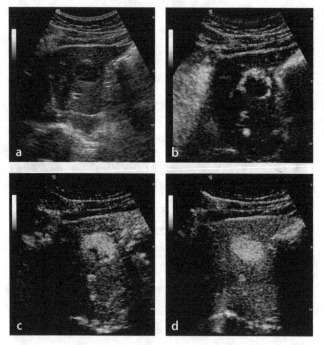

Fig. 9. Atypical hemangioma in a 25-year-old asymptomatic male. Rapid contrast filling during the arterial phase and long-lasting hyperenhancement. **a** Baseline, **b** Arterial phase (8s), **c** Arterial phase (20s), **d** Late phase (130s)

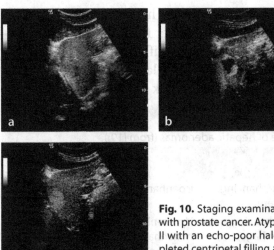

Fig. 10. Staging examination in a 69-year-old patient with prostate cancer. Atypical hemangioma in segment II with an echo-poor halo. Rapid arterial filling; completed centripetal filling after 2 min. **a** Baseline, **b** Arterial phase (17s), **c** Late phase (137s)

Hepatic Adenoma

Hepatic adenomas are rare and much more frequent in women [27] who are taking oral contraceptive medication. Patients with glycogen storage disease, hemochromatosis, and males using anabolic steroids may have an increased risk. Pregnancy may also be a risk factor [28]. There are two types of adenoma: one of bile duct and the other of liver-cell origin. The first is clinically irrelevant, as these adenomas stay very small and are incidentally detected by histology. The latter type contains hepatocysts that are capable of producing bile but lack bile ducts. Typically they also lack portal veins. US, CT, and MR findings frequently are nonspecific. Small adenomas are mostly missed on baseline US, larger ones often show hemorrhage. On baseline US, adenomas may be hypo-, iso- or hyperechoic. Most small adenomas are difficult to detect, as they have the same or similar B-mode characteristic as the surrounding tissue. In CEUS during arterial phase, some small peripheral arteries enhance before the liver tissue, and the tumor is quickly filled. During PV and late phase, the small, isoenhancing tumors disappear within the normal liver tissue. Larger adenomas often show hemorrhage (Table 5). Due to the small number of histologically proven cases of hepatic adenomas examined with CEUS, it is not clear whether this method can differentiate adenomas from FNH or highly differentiated HCC. Resection is always advocated in the case of a large hepatocellular adenoma (> 5 cm, Fig. 11) to reduce the risk of life-threatening rupture and malignant degeneration [29].

Table 5. CEUS appearance of hepatic adenomas (from [19])

Tumor entity	Arterial phase	PV phase	Delayed (late) phase
Typical features	Hyperenhancing, complete	Isoenhancing	Isoenhancing
Additional features	Nonenhancing areas (hemorrhage)	Hyperenhancing, nonenhancing areas (hemorrhage)	Nonenhancing central areas (hemorrhage)

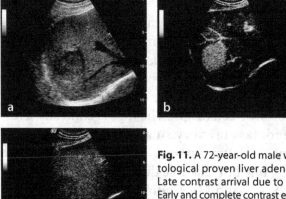

Fig. 11. A 72-year-old male with normal APF level. Histological proven liver adenoma (surgical specimen). Late contrast arrival due to pulmonary hypertension. Early and complete contrast enhancement and wash-out starting during PV phase suggested a malignant lesion. CT and MR (no fat tissue) could not confirm the diagnosis either. **a** Baseline, **b** Late arterial phase (29s), **c** Late phase (136s)

Focal Nodular Hyperplasia

With a prevalence of about 3%, FNH is the second most common tumor of the liver [2, 30]. Patients are typically in the second to fourth decade of life. FNH is a hyperplastic process of normal liver tissue components that have failed to build up a regular lobular architecture. It is a benign liver lesion, supplied by arteries without intratumoral shunts and containing normal hepatocytes, bile ducts, and RES (reticuloendothelial system). FNH contain Kupffer cells in varying numbers. Liver function tests are not affected. As the tumors are diagnosed much more frequently in women (female to male ratio 4:1), estrogens (including the use of oral contraceptives) and pregnancy are believed to play a pathogenetic role. We found FNH in males who were under anabolic medication or had a testicular tumor. It is now believed that FNH occurs as a result of a localized hepatocyte response to an underlying congenital arteriovenous malformation. Tumor growth and shrinkage may be affected by hormone status. At baseline US, FNH may show fibrous bands radiating from a central scar to the periphery. FNH has no capsule, and most present as iso- to slightly hyperechoic tumors. In fatty liver disease, FNH often presents as echo-poor lesions. Color Doppler findings may show a typical "spoke and wheel" sign of the supplying arteries. Spectral Doppler analysis can characterize the feeding artery as a low resistance vessel with a RI (resistive index) number around 0.51-0.58 [31, 32]. Large FHN may have more than one feeding artery that may also be located in the tumor periphery. Typically, FNH enhance very early (8-11 s, Figs. 12, 14, 15), and feeding and draining vessels can be seen. During the PV and late phases, they become iso/hyperenhancing. A central scar is not a specific sign, but can be found in up to 30% of patients (Table 6, Fig. 13).

Table 6. CEUS features in focal nodular hyperplasia (FNH) (from [19])

Tumor entity	Arterial phase	PV phase	Delayed (late) phase
Typical features	Hyperenhancing, complete	Hyperenhancing,	Iso-/hyperenhancing
Additional features	Early spoke and wheel sign, centrifugal filling, feeding artery	Hypoenhancing, central scar	Hypoenhancing, central scar

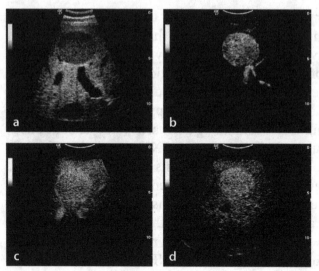

Fig. 12. Typical FNH, still hyperenhancing during late phase (**d**). **a** Baseline, **b** Arterial phase (18s), **c** PV phase (55s), **d** Late phase (3 min 7s)

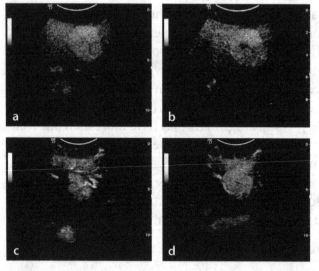

Fig. 13. Typical FNH, still hyperenhancing during late phase (**d**). Note the central scar. **a** Arterial phase (19s), **b** Arterial phase (21s), **c** PV phase (96s), **d** Late phase (159s)

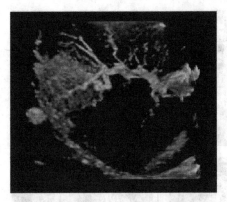

Fig. 14. Still image from 3-D contrast study (12-16s) of an FNH (segment IVa), demonstrating a ball of completely contrast-filled arteries and the supplying arteries. Accompanying the hepatic arteries, the central major portal-venous branches are already contrast-enhanced

We have observed three patients (two female, one male, all between 50 and 55 years) with histological proven FNH, which showed marked wash-out during PV and late phases. CT, MR, and, in one case, (Fig. 16) radionuclide scans were inconclusive as well.

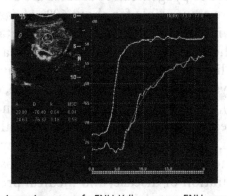

Fig. 15. Typical time-intensity curve of a FNH. *Yellow curve* = FNH, *green curve* = liver tissue

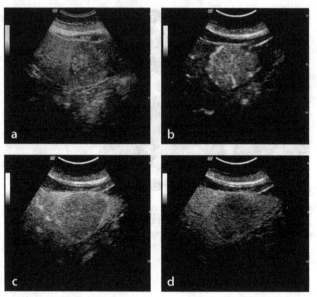

Fig. 16. Atypical FNH of the left liver lobe (tumor was surgically removed). A wash-out already starts during late arterial phase and is much more pronounced in later phases. **a** Baseline, **b** Arterial phase (14s), **c** PV phase (26s), **d** Late phase (135s)

Liver Abscess

The main source of pyogenic liver abscess are biliary-tract diseases, which are responsible for about 60% of cases. Infections from organs with venous drainage into the portal-venous system, mainly the digestive system, account for approximately one-fourth of liver abscesses. An infectious focus that spreads through the systemic circulation (for example, endocarditis, pyelonephritis), or compromised immunologic conditions (AIDS, malignant disease, or chemotherapy) may be other causes for liver abscesses. Contiguous spread from cholecystitis and the perihepatic space can result in a pyogenic liver abscess. Depending on size, duration of disease, and medical pretreatment, B-mode US shows great variability in the acoustic properties of the lesions. Internal septations or cavity debris may be detected. Gas bubbles may be found on the highest level of the abscess. On CEUS, a rim enhancement during arterial phase followed by a wash-out and sometimes a conversion to an echo-poor margin, indicates a focal edema. If liver parenchyma is destroyed, the enhancing septa are already filled during arterial phase and stay enhanced often until late phase (Table 7, Fig. 17). Due to the high arterial inflow, the abscess-carrying segment or liver lobe is often globally hyperenhancing as well.

Table 7. CEUS features in liver abscess (from [19])

Tumor entity	Arterial phase	PV phase	Delayed (late) phase
Typical features	Rim enhancement, no central enhancement	Hyper-, isoenhancing rim, no central enhancement	Hypoenhancing rim, no central enhancement
Additional features	Enhanced septa, hyperenhanced liver segment	Hypoenhancing, central scar rim, enhanced septa	

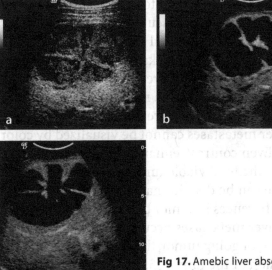

Fig 17. Amebic liver abscess in a 28-year-old patient from Afghanistan. **a** Baseline, **b** Arterial phase, **c** Late phase

Staging and Follow-Up of Patients with Metastatic Liver Disease

The liver is the second most common organ affected by metastatic disease, after the lymph nodes. Up to 80% of patients with extrahepatic malignancies will develop liver metastases during follow-up. At first staging examinations, 25-50% of patients prove to have liver metastases [33]. Multiple liver metastases (>90%) are much more common than solitary metastases (<10%). Both lobes are much more frequently involved (77%) than the right (20%) or left lobe (3%). The primary sites of tumors most commonly metastasizing to the liver are the eye and pancreas (70-75%), breast, gallbladder and extra hepatic bile ducts, colon or rectum (about 60%), and stomach (about 50%). Some 30% of metastatic lesions are < 10 mm in size. Even in patients with a malignancy, 80% of all lesions < 15 mm are benign [4].

In situ, tumors are avascular but not ischemic until they have reached the oxygen diffusion limit (up to 150-200 μm) from the nearest open host vessel [34]. The vascular network of a tumor may account for up to 10% of the total tumor volume. Due to their increased permeability, fluid leaks out of tumor vessels, causing an elevation in intratumoral pressure. The unenhanced central tumor area is much more likely to represent hypoxic tumor tissue than tumor necrosis. It is therefore not surprising, that the tumor network of liver metastases cannot be visualized by color Doppler techniques. Even contrast-enhanced CT or CEUS often does not demonstrate the total viable tumor tissue.

Normal liver tissue can be discriminated from abnormal tissue by imaging the differences in tumor blood supply: the nutrition of microscopic liver metastases occurs by diffusion or portal-venous supply. With ongoing tumor, the growing arterial supply dominates perfusion of the tumor [35].

With the exception of tiny lesions and the tumor periphery, there is no portal-venous supply. The small size of tumor microvessels (< 100 μm) precludes their direct visualization with CT, US, or angiography. In a few cases, intratumoral arteriovenous shunting may be present and has been described also by spectral Doppler examinations.

The recognition of a liver lesion as a metastatic focus significantly influences the patient's treatment and prognosis. Assessment of the number of metastases and their location is mandatory prior to surgery or ablation therapy and is needed to monitor chemotherapy as well. After detection and characterization of FLL, follow-up studies of metastatic liver disease are needed in order to monitor the response of the tumor burden to therapy. The vast majority of patients with metastatic liver disease are treated by chemotherapy. US is still one of the procedures that are frequently used in follow-up examinations. But due to changes in the acoustic properties of the surrounding liver tissue and the lesion itself, B-mode US has been reported to be inaccurate and thus is often not recommended [1].

Since the advent of US contrast agents, many studies have investigated the benefit of contrast media in detecting focal liver lesions – several of which especially focusing on the detection of malignant lesions. The presence and particularly the number and location of the liver lesions are important for planning interventional procedures or follow-up treatment.

The typical cause of enhancement in liver metastases reflects the arterial blood supply and the lack of portal-venous branches. A rather short time interval of arterial enhancement prior to liver tissue enhancement can be seen. It is followed by decreased enhancement during the PV phase and a mostly anechoic lesion during the late phase (Tables 8, 9).

Table 8. CEUS features in hypervascular liver metastases (from [19])

Tumor entity	Arterial phase	PV phase	Delayed (late) phase
Typical features	Hyperenhancement, complete	Hypoenhancing	Hypoenhancing, nonenhancing
Additional features	"Chaotic" vessels		

Table 9. CEUS features in hypovascular liver metastases (from [19])

Tumor entity	Arterial phase	PV phase	Delayed (late) phase
Typical features	Rim enhancement, complete	Hypoenhancing	Hypoenhancing, nonenhancing
Additional features	Complete enhancement, nonenhancing areas	Nonenhancing areas	

As in CT, CEUS metastases can present as hyper- or hypovascular lesions: Hypervascular tumors are characterized by an early arterial enhancement, which is present in most parts of the tumor. During PV phase, enhancement quickly decreases, and late phase shows hypoenhanced or nonenhanced lesion. For a few seconds between arterial and PV phase, isoenhancement may be seen. Thus, the arterial phase is the optimum phase for detection of these lesions, as the surrounding liver tissue enhances only minimally (Table 10, Fig. 18).

Table 10. Vascularization of liver metastases. Breast cancer, lymphomas, and melanomas may appear as hyper- or hypovascular

Hypervascular liver lesions	Hypovascular lesions
Neuroendocrine tumors (carcinoid)	Adenocarcinomas (GI tract, lung)
Islet cell tumors (insulinoma/gastrinoma)	Breast carcinoma
Chorioncarcinoma/ovarian cancer	Squamous cell carcinomas
Thyroid carcinoma	Lymphomas
Renal cell carcinoma	
Breast carcinoma	
Melanoma	
Sarcomas	
Lymphomas	

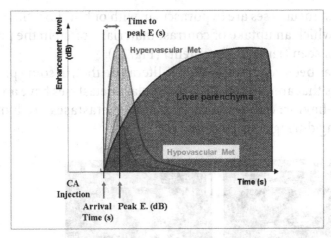

Fig. 18. Scheme of time-intensity curve between normal liver tissue, hyper-, and hypovascular liver metastases

The value of differentiating hyper- from hypovascular lesions is limited and can only offer hints regarding the suspected primary tumor. This approach may become more valuable in monitoring patients, as it reflects the vessel density, blood volume flow, and intratumoral pressure (Figs. 19, 20).

Fig. 19. Hypervascular liver metastases from ovarian cancer (**a**), carcinoid (**b**), renal cell carcinoma (central hypoxia/necrosis) (**c**), liposarcoma (3-D) (**d**)

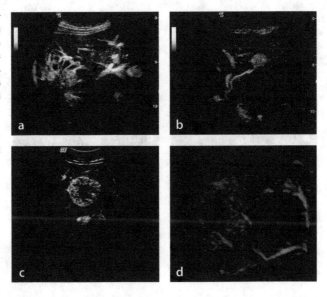

Most metastases are hypovascular, with only a short time interval in which an uptake of contrast material – often in the periphery – is seen (rim enhancement) (Fig. 21).

It has been reported in the CT literature that, in some primary tumors that are typically hypervascular, metastases have an atypical behavior: one-third of carcinoid metastases are hypoenhancing during arterial phase [9].

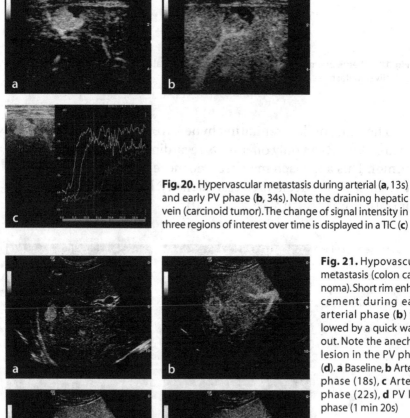

Fig. 20. Hypervascular metastasis during arterial (**a**, 13s) and early PV phase (**b**, 34s). Note the draining hepatic vein (carcinoid tumor). The change of signal intensity in three regions of interest over time is displayed in a TIC (**c**)

Fig. 21. Hypovascular metastasis (colon carcinoma). Short rim enhancement during early arterial phase (**b**) followed by a quick washout. Note the anechoic lesion in the PV phase (**d**). **a** Baseline, **b** Arterial phase (18s), **c** Arterial phase (22s), **d** PV late phase (1 min 20s)

Cystic metastases mostly come from mucin-producing colon or ovarian cancers, or represent regressive changes after chemotherapy.

In one study, liver metastases were correctly characterized in up to 95% of cases (204 out of 214 metastatic lesions) [15].

In many centers, CEUS has become the imaging technique of choice, especially in patients with a history of malignancies. For an experienced US examiner, CEUS is easy to learn and to interpret. Consequently, CEUS is a reliable diagnostic tool that improves diagnostic overall diagnostic accuracy. One center reported an improvement from about 50% in unenhanced baseline studies to about 88% during contrast examinations [36].

References

1. Giovagnoni A, Piga A, Argalia G et al (1993) Inadequacy of ultrasonography for monitoring response to treatment of liver metastases. J Clin Oncol 11(12):2451-2455
2. Karhunen PJ (1986) Benign hepatic tumours and tumour like conditions in men. J Clin Pathol 39:183-188
3. Jones EC, Chezmar JL, Nelson RC, Bernardino ME (1992) The frequency and significance of small (less than or equal to 15 mm) hepatic lesions detected by CT. AJR Am J Roentgenol 158(3):535-539
4. Schwartz LH, MD, Gandras EJ, Colangelo SM et al (1999) Prevalence and Importance of Small Hepatic Lesions Found at CT in Patients with Cancer. Radiology 210:71-74
5. Kinkel K, Lu Y, Both M et al (2002) Detection of hepatic metastases from cancers of the gastrointestinal tract by using noninvasive imaging methods (US, CT, MR imaging, PET): a meta-analysis. Radiology 224(3):748-756
6. Saini S (1997) Imaging of the hepatobiliary tract. N Engl J Med 336(26):1889-1894
7. Elias D, Sideris L, Pocard M et al (2005) Incidence of unsuspected and treatable metastatic disease associated with operable colorectal liver metastases discovered only at laparotomy (and not treated when performing percutaneous radiofrequency ablation). Ann Surg Oncol 12(4):298-302

8. Konopke R, Kersting S, Saeger HD, Bunk A (2005) Detection of liver lesions by contrast-enhanced ultrasound - comparison to intraoperative findings. Ultraschall Med 26(2):107-113
9. Paulson EK, McDermott VG, Keogan MT et al (1998) Carcinoid metastases to the liver: role of triple-phase helical CT. Radiology 206(1):143-150
10. Wilson SR, Burns PN, Muradali D et al (2000) Harmonic hepatic US with microbubble contrast agent: initial experience showing improved characterization of hemangioma, hepatocellular carcinoma, and metastasis. Radiology 215(1):153-161
11. Sahani DV, Kalva SP, Tanabe KK et al (2004) Intraoperative US in patients undergoing surgery for liver neoplasms: comparison with MR imaging. Radiology 232(3):810-814
12. Durand F, Regimbeau JM, Belghiti J et al (2001) Assessment of the benefits and risks of percutaneous biopsy before surgical resection of hepatocellular carcinoma. J Hepatol 35(2):254-258
13. Herszenyi L, Farinati F, Cecchetto A et al (1995) Fine-needle biopsy in focal liver lesions: the usefulness of a screening programme and the role of cytology and microhistology. Ital J Gastroenterol 27(9):473-478
14. Albrecht T, Hohmann J, Oldenburg A et al (2004) Detection and characterisation of liver metastases. Eur Radiol 14(Suppl 8):25-33
15. Solbiati L, Cova L, Kirn V, Tonolini M (2004) Contrast-enhanced sonography is highly reliable and potentially cost-effective for characterizing focal liver lesions initially detected by unenhanced sonography. RSNA, Chicago
16. von Herbay A, Vogt C, Willers R, Haussinger D (2004) Real-time imaging with the sonographic contrast agent SonoVue: differentiation between benign and malignant hepatic lesions. J Ultrasound Med 3(12):1557-1568
17. Bleuzen A, Tranquart F (2004) Incidental liver lesions: diagnostic value of cadence contrast pulse sequencing (CPS) and SonoVue. Eur Radiol 14(Suppl 8):53-62
18. Hohmann J, Skrok J, Puls R, Albrecht T (2003) Characterization of focal liver lesions with contrast-enhanced low MI real time ultrasound and SonoVue. Rofo 175(6):835-843
19. Albrecht T, Blomley M, Bolondi L et al (2004) Guidelines for the use

of contrast agents in ultrasound. January 2004. Ultraschall Med 25(4):249-256

20. Nelson RC, Chezmar JL (1990) Diagnostic approach to hepatic hemangiomas. Radiology 176(1):11-13

21. Leifer DM, Middleton WD, Teefey SA et al (2000) Follow-up of patients at low risk for hepatic malignancy with a characteristic hemangioma at US. Radiology 214(1):167-172

22. Caturelli E, Pompili M, Bartolucci F et al (2001) Hemangioma-like lesions in chronic liver disease: diagnostic evaluation in patients. Radiology 220(2):337-342

23. Brancatelli G, Federle MP, Blachar A, Grazioli L (2001) Hemangioma in the cirrhotic liver: diagnosis and natural history. Radiology 219(1):69-74

24. Vilgrain V, Boulos L, Vullierme MP et al (2000) Imaging of atypical hemangiomas of the liver with pathologic correlation. Radiographics 20(2):379-397

25. Ding H, Wang WP, Huang BJ et al (2005) Imaging of focal liver lesions: low-mechanical-index real-time ultrasonography with SonoVue. J Ultrasound Med 24(3):285-297

26. Reddy KR, Schiff ER (1993) Approach to a liver mass. Semin Liver Dis 13:423-435

27. Weimann A, Ringe B, Klempnauer J et al (1997) Benign liver tumors: differential diagnosis and indications for surgery. World J Surg 21(9):983-990

28. DeMenis E, Tramontin P, Conte N (1997) Successful resection of multifocal hepatic adenoma in pregnancy. South Medical Journal 22(8):357-361

29. Terkivatan T, de Wilt JH, de Man RA et al (2001) Indications and long-term outcome of treatment for benign hepatic tumors: a critical appraisal. Arch Surg 136(9):1033-1038

30. Ishak KG, Rabin L (1975) Benign tumors of the liver. Med Clin North Am 59:995-1013

31. Uggowitzer MM, Kugler C, Mischinger HJ et al (1999) Echo-enhanced Doppler sonography of focal nodular hyperplasia of the liver. J Ultrasound Med 18(7): 445-451; quiz 453-454

32. Wang Y, Wang WP, Ding H et al (2004) Resistance index in differential

diagnosis of liver lesions by color doppler ultrasonography. World J Gastroenterol 10(7):965-967

33. Edmunsen HA, Craig JR (1987) Neoplasms of the liver. In: Schiff L (ed) Diseases of the liver, 8th edn. Lippincott, Philadephia, p 1109
34. Folkman J, Beckner K (2000) Angiogenesis imaging. Acad Radiol 7(10):783-785
35. Baker ME, Paulson EK (1993) Hepatic metastatic disease. In: Meyers MA, (ed) Neoplasms of the digestive tract: imaging, staging, and management. Philadelphia, Lippincott-Raven, pp 361-395
36. Quaia E, Calliada F, Bertolotto M et al (2004) Characterization of focal liver lesions with contrast-specific US modes and a sulfur hexafluoride-filled microbubble contrast agent: diagnostic performance and confidence. Radiology 232(2):420-430

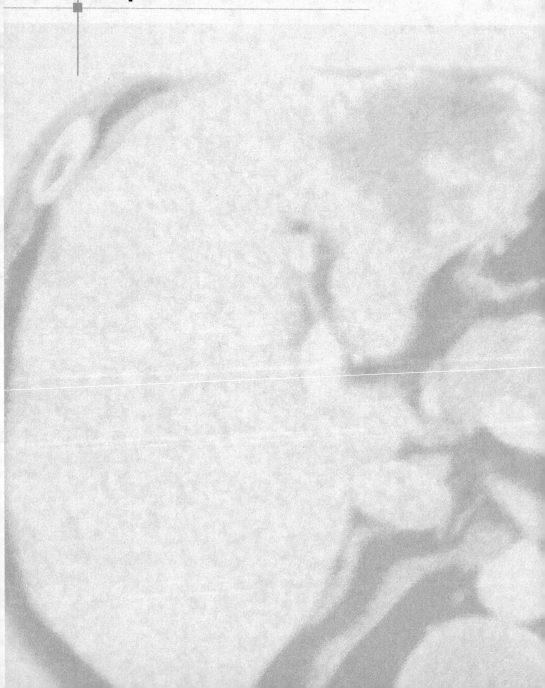

Jean-Michel Correas, Ahmed Khairoune,
Anais Vallet-Pichard,
Stanislas Pol, Olivier Hélénon

Chapter 3

Contrast-Enhanced Ultrasound in the Management of Cirrhotic Patients: HCC Diagnosis, Staging and Monitoring of Percutaneous Treatments

JEAN-MICHEL CORREAS[1], AHMED KHAIROUNE[1],
ANAIS VALLET-PICHARD[2],
STANISLAS POL[2], OLIVIER HÉLÉNON[1]
Department of Adult Radiology[1]
and Department of Hepatology[2]
Necker University Hospital, Paris, France

Introduction

Hepatocellular carcinoma (HCC) is the most frequent primary malignant liver tumor. In a vast majority of cases, it occurs in patients with chronic liver disease at the stage of cirrhosis. Its incidence is increasing in Western countries, ranging from 2.7 to 3.2 per 100000 [1]. This change is mainly due to the increasing incidence of chronic hepatitis C virus infection, while the incidence of cases attributed to alcoholic cirrhosis and chronic hepatitis B remains stable [2, 3]. Screening of HCC should focus on the population with the highest risk: chronic hepatitis B and C virus infection, alcohol abuse, cirrhosis irrespective of its etiology, male sex, and age over 55 years [3, 4]. The selection of patients for curative therapy is difficult. Surgical resection and liver transplantation still offer the best overall 5-year survival rate of approximately 30% [5]. However, only a limited number of patients, of less than 20%, can benefit from radical surgical treatments due to altered liver function and HCC extension and tumor volume. Percutaneous ablation using either ethanol injection or radiofrequency ablation (RFA) represents an alternative therapy to cure HCC when the number and size of the lesions is limited in Child A or B patients. Minimally invasive treatments can also be combined with chemoembolization. Their impact on HCC management will grow if the incidence of small lesions increases. Early detection of HCC is mandatory to benefit from the use of minimally invasive treatments such as RFA and to demonstrate an increase in survival rate. Chemoembolization and selective internal radiation therapy can be used in patients with large, infiltrative and /or multifocal lesions [6].

Detection of early HCC

The transformation of macroregenerative nodules to dysplastic lesions is characterized by the development of arterial neovascularization. This characteristic has become the basis for the detection and characterization of HCC using any imaging modality. Early detection of HCC remains a challenge in order to increase the number of patients that can benefit from curative therapy. It relies on the combination of serum α foeto-protein (AFP) levels and liver ultrasonography (US) that should be repeated each 4 to 6 months [7]. However, these two screening tests have many limitations due to their limited sensitivity. They are still used in most cases because of their low cost and lack of morbidity. Serum AFP sensitivity and positive predictive value are low, ranging from 39% to 64% and 9% to 32%, respectively [8, 9]. An increase in AFP is not specific for HCC and serum AFP levels remain normal in almost 50% of HCC below 3 cm in diameter. The sensitivity of US examination is limited, ranging from 40% to 70% for lesions below 2 cm in diameter. In cirrhotic patients its sensitivity can reach 78%, with a specificity of 93% and a positive predictive value of 73% [8]. Two conditions must be met to detect a nodule by US: first, the US beam should reach the nodule, and secondly, the ultrasonic properties of the nodule should be different from the surrounding cirrhotic parenchyma. The liver atrophy and the interposition of bowel gases reduce the accessibility of the liver parenchyma. The distortion and attenuation of the US beam due to fibrosis, steatohepatitis and micro/macronodules limits the study of deep parts of the liver. In macronodular cirrhosis, the correct identification of HCCs below 2 cm becomes extremely difficult due to the large number of regenerating nodules and the lack of specific features at baseline US.

Small HCC can appear as a hypo-, iso- or hyperechoic mass and cannot be distinguished from macroregenerative nodules and dysplastic lesions. Color Doppler US might be useful for the characterization of focal liver lesions in cirrhosis, as most of HCCs exhibit arterial Doppler signals [10, 11]. Color and Power Doppler US can increase US accuracy for the characterization of HCC. However, the clinical value of this feature remains limited as Doppler signals are frequently attenuated by the cirrhotic liver. Thus, deep and small HCC will not exhibit arterial signals in most cases.

■ Contrast-Enhanced US

Contrast-enhanced US (CEUS) of the liver at low acoustic power became available with the introduction of ultrasound contrast agents (USCAs) containing microbubbles filled with perfluorocarbon gases, such as sulfur hexafluoride (SonoVue®, Bracco, Milan, Italy). These USCAs are pure blood flow agents with a good tolerance in clinical practice. Low mechanical index (MI) imaging techniques allow continuous detection of the microbubbles during all phases of their liver transit, including arterial, portal and delayed phases. Hepatocellular lesions exhibit specific kinetics in more than 95% of the cases, with a strong enhancement during the arterial phase followed by a rapid wash-out [12-15]. During the delayed phase, they are usually echo-poor compared to the surrounding parenchyma, except for well-differentiated lesions that can remain isoechoic (Figs. 1, 2). Approximately 70% of HCCs will become hypoechoic during late phase imaging, depending upon cellular differentiation [16]. The hypoechogenic pattern during late phase is less marked and can be very limited, at the contrary of the one observed for metastases. The performance of CEUS for detection

Fig. 1a-f. Child A cirrhosis in a 67-year-old woman with chronic hepatitis C virus infection, previously treated for a unique HCC by RFA 3 years before. The liver is strongly attenuating the signal. **a** US examination detected a 2-cm hypoechoic nodule in the upper segment IV. **b** Color Doppler US did not reveal any abnormal flow. **c-e** Contrast-enhanced US was performed using "Vascular Rendering Imaging" after a bolus injection of 2.4 ml of SonoVue® (Bracco, Italy). With this modality, microbubbles in the capillaries are colorized in yellow. During arterial phase, the lesion poorly enhanced but the increased vascularity became obvious (**c**, *white arrow*). This modality allows separation of the perfusion information (**d**) from the anatomic information (**e**). This feature is crucial during the review of the cineloop to precisely identify the area of enhancement. **f** CT did not detect any enhancement of the focal mass. However, biopsy performed during RF ablation confirmed the presence of a poorly differentiated HCC. In this case CEUS sensitivity for the detection of vascularity was superior to that of CT

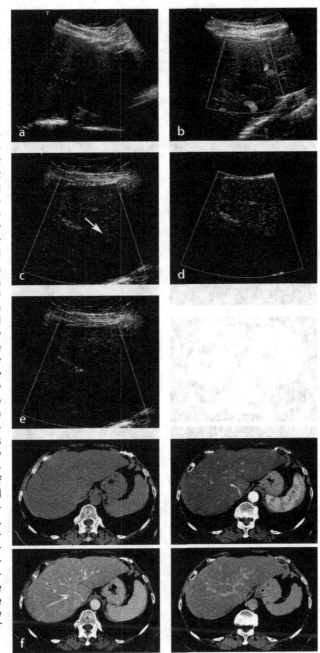

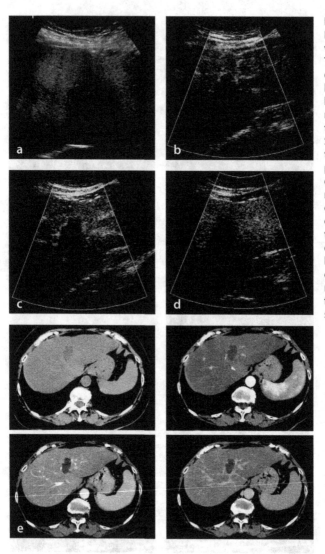

Fig. 2a-e. Monitoring of RF ablation of HCC 6 weeks after treatment. The lesion is the one described in Fig. 1. **a** The lesion appeared slightly heterogeneous on B mode. **b-d** CEUS with VRI technique following SonoVue® administration at arterial phase (**b**), portal phase (**c**) and delayed phase (**d**) did not reveal persistence of enhancement. The ablated area covered entirely the site of the previously detected nodule. The lesion was considered as correctly treated with no residual tumor. **e** CT confirmed the lack of persisting tumor of HCCs can be improved if they can be detected not only during arterial phase but also during the prolonged late phase (Figs. 3, 4). Development of specific imaging techniques and USCA with different properties should be directed to increase the impact of CEUS in cirrhosis. Indeed, the short duration of the arterial phase is an inherent limitation to CEUS for the detection of small HCCs. The total USCA dose can be fractioned to obtain repeated arterial phases. The reproducibility of the USCA effect should be maintained over the duration of the examination. In practice, no more than 2 to 3 arterial phases can be obtained with available USCAs. New approaches using USCA with specific uptake into the reticuloendothelial system might increase the rate of HCC with hypoechoic appearance during late phase. The frequency of the hypoechoic pattern during late phase is also dependent upon the specific US imaging modality. The most recent techniques using simultaneous modulation of phase and amplitude, such as Cadence Contrast Pulse sequencing technology (Siemens-Acuson, Mountain View, CA), are very promising [15].

The typical kinetics of HCC at CEUS are almost similar to those of other imaging techniques such as contrast-enhanced CT and MRI. This similarity should be helpful for the diffusion of the CEUS out of experts' hands.

US contrast enhancement kinetics also provide information that allows characterization of other focal liver lesions that can be found in cirrhotic patients, such as regenerating and dysplastic nodules and hemangiomas. The differential diagnosis between regenerating nodules and HCC becomes easy as they do not exhibit any strong enhancement during the arterial phase, but they enhance simultaneously to the surrounding nontumoral parenchyma. They typically disappear during portal and delayed phases. High-grade dysplastic nodules can exhibit some enhancement during the arterial phase or appear hypoechoic during the delayed phase. It does not seem critical to differentiate them from HCCs as they can be considered as premalignant lesions [16]. Low-grade dysplastic nodules behave as regenerative nodules. Hemangiomas represent the most common solid benign lesion in the normal population and are rarely found in cirrhotic patients. Their hyperechoic pattern is unusual

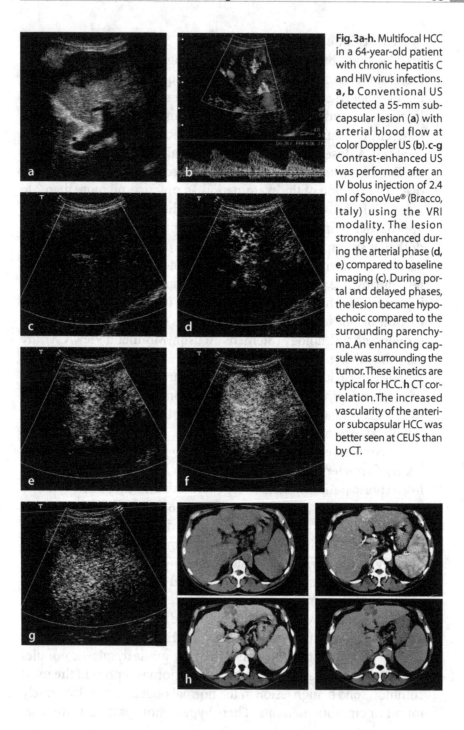

Fig. 3a-h. Multifocal HCC in a 64-year-old patient with chronic hepatitis C and HIV virus infections. **a, b** Conventional US detected a 55-mm subcapsular lesion (**a**) with arterial blood flow at color Doppler US (**b**). **c-g** Contrast-enhanced US was performed after an IV bolus injection of 2.4 ml of SonoVue® (Bracco, Italy) using the VRI modality. The lesion strongly enhanced during the arterial phase (**d, e**) compared to baseline imaging (**c**). During portal and delayed phases, the lesion became hypoechoic compared to the surrounding parenchyma. An enhancing capsule was surrounding the tumor. These kinetics are typical for HCC. **h** CT correlation. The increased vascularity of the anterior subcapsular HCC was better seen at CEUS than by CT.

Fig. 4a-c. In the same patient as in Fig. 3, an additional small HCC was also detected in between segment III and II. This lesion was not seen on baseline imaging even during the review of the cineloops acquired during the examination. **a, b** The lesion strongly enhanced during arterial phase (**a**, *arrow*) and became hypoechoic during late phase (**b**). **c** CT confirmed the presence of this typical HCC

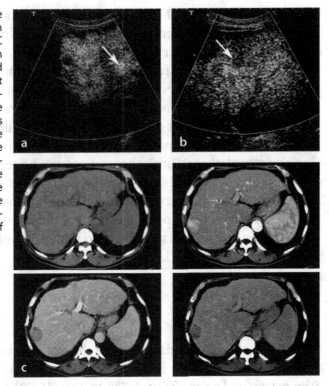

in this patient population, where any focal lesion over 2 cm should be considered as a potential HCC. They typically do not show any vascularity at color Doppler US. However, they exhibit a very specific pattern of enhancement with peripheral globular or rim-like enhancement during arterial phase. During portal phase, they tend to fill with centripetal enhancement pattern, but complete filling may not occur event after a long waiting period [17]. This difference from CT and MR results from the lack of interstitial diffusion of the compound and the short duration of the microbubbles. Hemangiomas will become iso-or hyperechoic during late phase. Small hypervascular hemangiomas can be difficult to distinguish from HCC as they enhance intensively during arterial phase without a peripheral globular pattern. In this case, the presence of a hypoechoic appearance during late phase strongly suggests the presence of HCC. If the lesion remains isoechoic, it cannot be differentiated from a small HCC and MRI should be used to distinguish these two lesions. Well-differentiated HCCs are more difficult to diagnose because the hypervascular pattern can be missing [16]. Peripheral cholangiocarcinomas can also be found in cirrhotic patients. At baseline, these lesions are usually hypo- or isoechoic, depending on the cirrhotic liver. The margins are irregular and color Doppler US cannot detect intratumoral vascularity. At CEUS, most cholangiocarcinomas do not exhibit a hypervascular pattern during arterial phase. Rim enhancement can be seen during portal phase. Hypervascular cholangiocarcinomas exhibit a very transient arterial enhancement and become strongly hypoechoic during late phase, with no enhancement of the fibrotic components of the lesion due to the lack of extravascular microbubbles at the contrary of CT and MRI.

■ CEUS Performance

CEUS is an effective modality for the characterization of focal liver lesions, and particularly for HCC, with a sensitivity ranging from 92% to 94% and a specificity of 87% to 96% [16-20]. USCAs increase the detection of HCCs with a high sensitivity (above 95%) and specificity (85%). The efficacy of CEUS for the detection of HCC hypervascularity is superior to CT [20, 21]. In HCCs below 2 cm in diameter, only 54-61% of the lesions appears hypervascular at CEUS, but this number is greater compared to CT (43-49%) (Figs.1, 3). In larger HCCs, the rate of hypervascular lesions increases up to 91-97% at CEUS and 76-87% at CT. Hypovascular HCCs remain as an issue as they can easily be missed during both arterial and portal phases. They can represent up to 8% of HCCs below 3 cm [21].

CEUS also contributes to the staging of HCCs as tumor thrombus typically exhibits a strong enhancement during the arterial phase in contrast to bland thrombus.

CEUS can also improve the percutaneous placement of needles or electrodes [22]. After ablation using percutaneous ethanol injection or radiofrequency application, CEUS is the imaging modality of choice in order to assess immediate (Fig. 5) and delayed therapeutic efficacy (Fig. 2) [23, 24]. It allows immediate repositioning of the electrodes in case of incomplete treatment. Per-procedural CEUS reduces the rate of partial necrosis from 16.1% to 5.1% in experienced hands [24].

Clinical Management of HCC with and without the Use of USCA

The clinical management of HCC was discussed at the EASL meeting in Barcelona, depending on the size of the nodule at US and serum AFP levels [7]. Four situations were found without the use of ultrasound contrast media. (1) If US failed to detect a nodule while serum AFP levels are increasing, a contrast-enhanced helical CT (CE-CT) is needed to rule out an HCC. (2) When a nodule smaller than 1 cm is detected at conventional US, the US examination should be repeated after 3 months, because almost 50% of small nodules are likely to be HCCs. (3) When the nodule is between 1 and 2 cm in diameter, noninvasive criteria have been proposed: two different imaging techniques exhibiting for this lesion arterial enhancement as a reflect of the increased vascularity of the tumor, or a single imaging technique demonstrating arterial enhancement and AFP levels higher than 400 ng/ml. Biopsy might be still considered in patients who cannot benefit from liver transplantation. (4) In patients with a nodule above 2 cm in diameter, a CE-CT or CE-MRI is needed to characterize the nodule.

The algorithm from the EASL can be revisited to define new indications for CEUS. In the first situation of rising AFP without any focal liver mass detected at conventional US, CEUS can be proposed to improve the detection of HCC. However, the shortness of the arterial phase, while the entire liver is scanned, remains a limitation. In the second situation of a nodule smaller than 1 cm detected at conventional US, CEUS can be performed immediately in order to characterize the lesion. If a hypervascular pattern is detected, the diagnosis of small HCC will be confirmed

Fig. 5a-g. Monitoring of RF ablation of HCC (same patient as in Fig. 3). The CE-US is performed 15 min after the end of the RF procedure. **a** The cool-tip cluster electrode was placed within the 55-mm tumor using an approach parallel to the anterior capsule to avoid direct puncture of the lesion. **b, c** The lesion was surrounded by a hyperechoic attenuating halo at the end of the RFA procedure (**b**). Fifteen minutes later, most of the macrobubbles have disappeared (**c**). Color Doppler US did not reveal any flow within the ablated area. **d-f** At baseline VRI imaging (**d**), no artifact was noted that could be attributed to the presence of residual macrobubbles. After injection of SonoVue®, the lesion was studied during the arterial portal and delayed phases. The procedure was apparently successful. The ablated area seemed homogeneous without residual tumor (**e**). However, a careful review of the cineloop during the arterial phase revealed the persistence of a rim of strongly enhancing tissues (**f**, *arrow*). **g** CT confirmed the presence of a small enhancing area (*arrow*). The ablation should be considered as incomplete. However, no additional ablation was considered, and further treatment consisted in chemoembolization

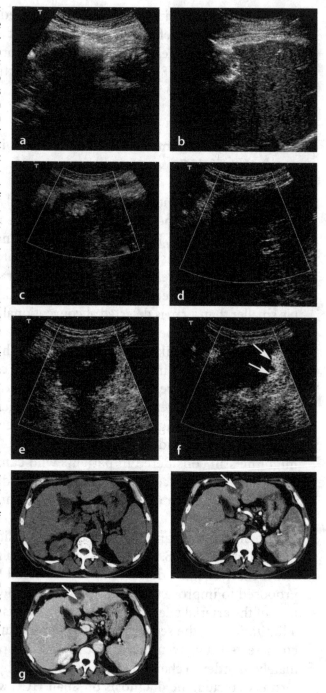

by a second imaging modality. Compared to the conventional algorithm, this approach will reduce the delay for treatment. The follow-up might be improved because the risk of losing the patient is reduced. In the third situation of a 1- to 2-cm nodule, CEUS should become one of the two techniques for the demonstration of arterial enhancement. In case of discrepancy between CT and MRI, CEUS might be superior as it allows continuous monitoring of the enhancement. The purely intravascular location of the microbubbles can also explain the superiority of CEUS in difficult cases. In the fourth situation of a nodule above 2 cm in diameter, CEUS can be used to characterize the lesion, particularly if CT or MRI cannot be performed. Additional indications are for percutaneous ablation, optimal lesion targeting in case of poor visibility, immediate assessment for the detection of incomplete treatment leading to repositioning the electrode during the same procedure (Fig. 5) and long-term follow-up (Fig. 2). The screening of cirrhotic patients using CEUS remains to be evaluated in larger studies, as well as its pharmacoeconomic impact. However, CEUS might increase the sensitivity of US, as demonstrated in a limited series of 48 patients where the detection rate was 88%, despite the small size of the lesions (70% below 2 cm in diameter) [25].

New algorithms should be developed to take into account the role of CEUS. However, the imaging technique is evolving very quickly and results between series are not easily comparable. The problem of truly hypovascular HCCs persists particularly in nodules of 1 to >2 cm. If a hypervascular pattern is detected by CEUS (even if missed by CT or MRI), an aggressive policy should be proposed that includes liver biopsy [21].

References

1. Bosch FX, Ribes J (2000) Epidemiology of liver cancer in Europe. Can J Gastroenterol 14:621-630
2. El-Serag HB, Mason AC (2000) Risk factors for the rising rates of primary liver cancer in the United States. Arch Intern Med 160:3227-3230
3. Bruix J, Llovet JM (2002) Prognostic prediction and treatment strategy in hepatocellular carcinoma. Hepatology 35:519-524
4. Benvegnu L, Fattovich G, Noventa F et al (1994) Concurrent hepatitis B and C virus infection and risk of hepatocellular carcinoma in cirrhosis. A prospective study. Cancer 74:2442-2448
5. Schwartz SI, Spencer FC, Galloway AC et al (1999) Liver. In: Principles of surgery. 7th ed. New York, NY: McGraw-Hill, pp 1410-1411
6. Clark HP, Carson WF, Kavanagh PV et al (2005) Staging and current treatments of hepatocellular carcinoma. Radiographics 25:S3-S23
7. Bruix J, Sherman M, Llovet JM et al (2001) EASL Panel of Experts on HCC. Clinical management of hepatocellular carcinoma. Conclusions of the Barcelona-2000 EASL conference. European Association for the Study of the Liver. J Hepatol 35:421-430
8. Pateron D, Ganne N, Trinchet JC et al (1994) Prospective study of screening for hepatocellular carcinoma in Caucasian patients with cirrhosis. J Hepatol 20:65-71
9. Oka H, Tamori A, Kuroki T et al (1994) Prospective study of alpha-fetoprotein in cirrhotic patients monitored for development of hepatocellular carcinoma. Hepatology 19:61-66
10. Tanaka S, Kitamura T, Fujita M et al (1990) Color Doppler flow imaging of liver tumors. AJR Am J Roentgenol 154:509-514
11. Lencioni R, Pinto F, Armillotta N, Bartolozzi C (2001) Assessment of tumour vascularity in hepatocellular carcinoma: comparison of power Doppler US and color Doppler US. Radiology 201:353-358
12. Leen E (2001) The role of contrast-enhanced ultrasound in the characterisation of focal liver lesions. Eur Radiol 11:E27-34
13. Fracanzani AL, Burdick L, Borzio M et al (2001) Contrast-enhanced Doppler ultrasonography in the diagnosis of hepatocellular carcinoma and premalignant lesions in patients with cirrhosis. Hepatology 34:1109-1112

14. Tranquart F, Bleuzen A, Correas JM et al (2003) Contrast ultrasound imaging in liver disease. J Radiol 84:2025-2040

15. Nicolau C, Vilana R, Bru C (2004) The use of contrast-enhanced ultrasound in the management of the cirrhotic patient and for detection of HCC. Eur Radiol 14[8]:P63-71

16. Nicolau C, Catala V, Vilana R (2004) Evaluation of Hepatocellular carcinoma using Sonovue, a second generation ultrasound contrast agent: correlation with cellular differentiation. Eur Radiol 14:1092-1099

17. Tranquart F, Bleuzen A (2004) Incidental liver lesions: diagnostic value of cadence contrast pulse sequencing (CPS) and SonoVue. Eur Radiol 14[8]:P53-62

18. Wen YL, Kudo M, Zheng RQ et al (2004) Characterization of hepatic tumors: value of contrast-enhanced coded phase-inversion harmonic angio. AJR Am J Roentgenol 182:1019-1026

19. Tanaka S, Ioka T, Oshikawa O et al (2001) Dynamic sonography of hepatic tumors. AJR Am J Roentgenol 177:799-805

20. Giorgio A, Ferraioli G, Tarantino L (2004) Contrast-enhanced sonographic appearance of hepatocellular carcinoma in patients with cirrhosis: comparison wit-h contrast-enhanced helical CT appearance. AJR Am J Roentgenol 183:1319-1326

21. Bolondi L, Gaiani S, Celli N et al (2005) Characterization of small nodules in cirrhosis by assessment of vascularity: the problem of hypovascular hepatocellular carcinoma. Hepatology 42:27-34

22. Skjoldbye B, Pedersen MH, Struckmann J et al (2002) Improved detection and biopsy of solid liver lesions using pulse-inversion ultrasound scanning and contrast agent infusion. Ultrasound Med Biol 28:439-444

23. Numata K, Isozaki T, Ozawa Y et al (2003) Percutaneous ablation therapy guided by contrast-enhanced sonography for patients with hepatocellular carcinoma. AJR Am J Roentgenol 180:143-149

24. Solbiati L, Tonolini M, Cova L (2004) Monitoring RF ablation. Eur Radiol 14[8]:P34-42

25. Solbiati L, Tonolini M, Cova L, Goldberg SN (2001) The role of contrast-enhanced ultrasound in the detection of focal liver lesions. Eur Radiol 11:E15-26